MAN, DOG, STROKE

MAN, DOG, STROKE

Musings of a Deeside Whippet and his Master

Eric Sinclair

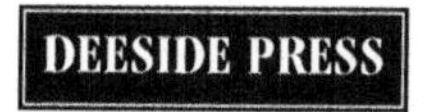

First published in the United Kingdom in 2011
by Deeside Press

ISBN 978-0-9570995-0-0

Proceeds from the sale of this book will be donated by the author to The Stroke Association, a UK-wide charity whose vision is a world where there are fewer strokes and all those touched by stroke get the help they need.

Produced by
The Choir Press, Gloucester

Contents

La vie doit avoir un courant, l'eau qui ne coule
pas se corrompt

(Alphonse de Lamartine)

*(Life should have a current, water which does not
flow becomes stagnant)*

1

A Christmas to forget

Unconditional love, anyone?

When I first meet new dogs and new humans I usually try to give the "to know me is to love me" look. Let me try to describe it for you. Brown eyes gaze up at you soulfully out of a long mournful face. Ears are slightly cocked. The head is held at a wistful angle. There may be a twitch of the tail. There is a longing in that look for love and food – not necessarily in that order. Have you got the picture? I'm pretty good at this look because I'm a fairly thin, rather handsome silver-brindle whippet with a long white mournful face and a white chest of manly proportions. "To know me is to love me" has got me many a meaty treat.

But, bones and biscuits, nothing, and I mean *nothing*, could have persuaded me to put on that look first thing on Christmas morning last December.

I thought I had sussed Christmas. There's a lot of human excitement, including much noisy rushing around by small children. There's lots of interesting rustling as parcels are opened. Sometimes the contents give off a fine soapy smell and there's always a generous whiff of cooking food in the background. I know that I just have to wait patiently until the humans have finished exploring their rustling parcels and have done with all the kissing and calling out that they do, and have got a bit bored with their toys. Then the moment will come when they remember that I, Hamish, loving and faithful family dog throughout the year, am now due the chance to tear into my very own Christmas present.

There's always a faint scent of dog about my present when Master or Mistress hands it to me. I give one of my rare yelps of delight then tear into it without delay (I don't *do* delay), tossing the shreds of paper to one side and biting into the toy squeaky thing or chewy bone hidden within them – squeaks and bones are about the extent of Master's imagination and I happen to know it's Master who always buys my present. Mistress says he spoils me.

Anyway, this Christmas it wasn't like that.

I woke up on Christmas morning feeling as rough as a dog who's been dragged through a nest of kittens. My tummy had swollen to twice its usual size and the pain just throbbed and throbbed. I couldn't even haul myself in the direction of breakfast. As for Christmas presents or squeaks or bones, I couldn't face any of them. I lay in my kitchen bed panting slightly. I was not a well dog.

It was Mistress who first noticed my plight and

communicated her disapproval of my swollen state with a single – and distinctly un-Christmassy – "Tut!"

Not a present had been opened, and the next thing I knew was that Master was standing over me in his ruffled early morning state. Master's early morning appearance has been the subject of many jokes over the years, but I could tell no-one was joking this time. It was then that Master uttered the V word. "I really think we should call the V**," said Master. Sometimes he teases me about this – but this time I knew he was serious. "On Christmas Day?" said Mistress. "That'll cost an arm and a leg." This is one human expression I've never understood, but it didn't seem to have any effect on Master, who was starting to stroke my head and tickle me behind the ears. He looked me directly in the face and I swear I could see moisture in his eyes. Biscuits and treats, my stomach was now aching really badly and if the V** could make it better, then so be it. I slumped back in my bed thinking of Master's moist eyes.

The next few hours are now a blur to me, but I know it was icy cold outside and I was taken a long way in the car bed before I was carried outside by Mistress and staggered with her into the house of an unknown She-V**. She prodded every part of me, plunged a nippy needle in my neck and handed Mistress a box of pills that rattled in a rather interesting way. Then I slept and slept and slept and forgot all about Christmas bones and squeaks. Days passed during which Mistress fed me the pills wrapped in bits of cake. Humans came to and from the house enjoying Christmas and New Year and parties. I wasn't in the mood for any of it.

Finally, I had another visit to the V** – this time the known V**. The known V**'s house has a scent of tense dogs and suffering cats. I don't mind the suffering cats, but I hardly had time to think of that on this visit. The known V** put me to sleep and, when I woke up, I had one of those horrible plastic lampshades over my head. I staggered a bit, but I had no more pain!

Just before we left the V**'s house, Master did what he always does on such occasions. He took out a black pouch and took a shiny card from it. The V** has a machine which half eats this card. Master sighs, as if he is sorry for the shiny plastic card, and, after a while, he punches the V**'s machine with his fingers four times. Then the V**'s machine releases Master's shiny card and Master slips it back into the black pouch and into his pocket. I've never understood this process, but I sense that Master is not enjoying himself while it is happening.

It was some time after this, back home, that Master sat down and gave me the Chat. He had the shiny plastic card in his hand and a sombre look on his face. I decided it was time for the "To know me is to love me" look – which I could manage, even with the lampshade on my head – and while Master spoke, I gave him the look, stared at the shiny plastic card, and listened carefully to the Chat. "Hamish," Master said, "Your illness has punished this card harder than it has ever been punished before. You are now starting to get better and it will have been worthwhile if you live for another few years."

I thought "Am I not more important than your shiny plastic card? How can I make myself live for another few years? How can Master say these things?" Sausages and bones, these are big questions for a dog.

The questions were so big and so tiring to think of that I dropped the look, lay down and fell asleep. As I dozed, I dreamed again of Christmas morning. I dreamed of the terrible pain and remembered the moisture in Master's eyes. Then somehow I knew there was more to Master's words than the plastic card and the punishment it had suffered. Those moist eyes clinched it – I felt happy and secure.

Unconditional love, anyone? I'll keep you posted.

2

The Rica Hotel

The Rica Hotel is an unlikely setting for a life-changing experience.

The hotel lies a few miles outside Oslo, close to the city's Gardermoen Airport. It is an unremarkable modern building set within one of those typical featureless areas of commercial warehousing, hotels and light industrial sites, which lie beside many of the world's airports. Having taken a train from Bergen that morning, I checked into the Rica Hotel on 16 July 2004 with the help of my son, Iain, who was working at the nearby Miklagard Golf Course.

On the 17 July, we took a train into town, strolled round central Oslo and climbed to the top of the Olympic ski jump to view a wide panorama of the city, its harbour and nearby islands. It was a bright sunny ordinary day and we sat for a while in a harbour-side open air restaurant enjoying a drink, some over- priced food, some renewed family bonding. Iain pointed out the bars and clubs where he and some of his work colleagues had spent nights out together. We watched a large white cruise liner edging her way regally out of the harbour, slowly gathering speed as she wound her way out into the Baltic. We paused at a spot where pavement artists were sketching portraits of tourists – they had attracted quite a crowd of locals and visitors. We took a train back from Oslo Central station and ate at a restaurant in Jessheim, close to where Iain lived. Afterwards, he dropped me off at the hotel and we agreed to meet again the following morning for a round of golf. As he drove off, I cursed myself for forgetting to get a note of his new mobile phone number. Too bad, I'd get it tomorrow.

It was my wedding anniversary next day, and before going to bed, I made a mental note to give my wife, Jo, a call the following morning. As a man, self-evidently I needed to underline this message to myself, so I laid my mobile phone on a table beside my bed. Although it was about 10 p.m. the Norwegian summer sun was still bright outside as I closed the curtains.

So drew to a close the last normal day of my life.

The following day I wakened at about 7 a.m. I tried to sit up; however, an invisible but powerful vice seemed to be pinning me to the bed. My face felt oddly tight and my left arm as though an electrical current was silently surging through it. I was briefly reminded of the Kafka novel (What was its name?) where a young man awakens to find he has been transformed into a giant insect, which, because it is on its back, can only wave its legs feebly in the air. The trouble was I didn't seem to be able to move my legs or arms at all. With growing fright and disbelief I tried to roll over. My heart seemed to be racing in an alarming way and my next thought as I gradually became more conscious of the all-pervading weakness in my body was that I must be having a heart attack. With a further lurch to the left I found myself precariously close to the edge of the large double bed. I gazed around the room as far as I could. Everything seemed exactly as it had been the night before – television in the corner, suitcase on a rack beside one wall, socks, underpants, leather rucksack close to the bed on the floor, shoes casually placed next to it.

I fell rather than slid off the bed on to the carpet with the thud of a dead weight and started to review my position. Prone on the floor, I tentatively explored my loss of power. My heart was racing and I could feel its beat against the floor. I was lying heavily – unusually heavily, I thought – on my left side. I realised that I could not move my left leg, nor could I move my left arm, which was now stretched out at an odd angle. I felt no pain at all which surely seemed to make it unlikely that I was in the throes of a heart attack. One side of my face felt strangely tight and numb, as if it had been anaesthetised by a dentist. The anaesthetic, however, would have had to be unusually extensive and cruel in its reach as the area of tight numbness appeared to reach from the top of my scalp to the lower jaw on the left side of my face.

I found it difficult to grasp the comprehensive

destruction which appeared to have been wreaked on my body.

The left hand side of my face was lying numbly on the carpet and I felt an almost irresistible desire to shut my eyes, go to sleep and reawaken in a sane world where this awful event had not happened. Perhaps I did drift off for a few moments. When I next consciously examined my predicament, nothing had changed. I appeared to be still alive. My heart was still racing with shock and fear. My body seemed as powerless and weak as before. I also seemed to be desperate to pee. I tried to struggle upright once again but could not stir from where I was lying.

I became aware that my head was lying very close to the bedside table. I remembered that I'd left the mobile phone on this table – I could phone Jo – not quite the anniversary greeting I'd intended, but contact with someone who could definitely speak English and with whom I could share my predicament. Instinctively, before I picked up the phone I tried my voice, whispering "hello" to the empty darkened room with a strange, weak sound that seemed wholly detached from my own voice. With my right hand I switched on the phone. Reassuringly the dial lit up in its normal pale blue and asked me to key in my personal code. Everything was not crazy because I could remember the code and typed it in awkwardly – 5555.

It took a few seconds for the phone to come fully to life and a further few seconds for me to press "Home" and to connect with the familiar UK ringing sound. It was only when Jo's sleepy voice answered that I realised the enormity of what I was doing to her. It was our anniversary. Norway was an hour ahead of UK time. She was still in bed. She had probably been asleep. A picture of our bedroom with its coombed ceilings, early morning light and drawn curtains flashed through my mind. "Jo!" I slurred, summoning up as much voice as I could, "something awful has happened to my body. I can't seem to stand up. Can you contact Iain and ask him to come to the hotel." Even as I said this, I was beginning to think of the time it would all take. Could I wait that long? I rang off, leaving her to contact Iain. I learned later that the only words Jo understood from my message were "Contact Iain". The rest was an incoherent jumble. I lay and waited. Perhaps I could call an ambulance. I just wanted some qualified person to tell me what was wrong. With another struggle I keyed in 112. Almost immediately a Norwegian voice crackled at the other end. With all the strength I could muster, I croaked, "Doctor. I need a doctor. Room 103. Rica Hotel. Gardermoen."

A few moments later – or it might have been much longer, for I appeared to awaken from sleep – the hotel receptionist was standing beside me. From where I lay, she seemed impossibly tall and far away. My pyjama-clad body felt vulnerable and undignified.

"Are you ill?" she asked. Then, before I could reply, added, "The ambulance you called will soon be here."

So things were happening. Somewhere a system was springing into action. I lay back on the carpet. I feared that I must be dying. I felt weak, ill, tired and no longer in control. A great wave of regret and emotion engulfed me and I thought of things I would never see or do again. I was sobbing uncontrollably, thinking of our home in the Glen Dye forest, of Jo, wakened by a crazy telephone call and now worried about what might be happening. I wanted to speak to her and tell her everything was okay. In reality, I was convinced that I was dying, that my face on a rough Norwegian hotel carpet would be my final living sensation. I was experiencing what it was like to confront death, and was not proud of the fear and regret I felt.

The door was pushed open and two green-uniformed paramedics stood over me. They were asking questions, but I was able only to weep. It didn't seem to matter. They were gently sliding me on to a stretcher. More disturbance and Iain was in the room, pale and drained. Like the receptionist he seemed impossibly tall and far away. I seemed unable to communicate other than with tears.

The paramedics expertly slid my stretcher on to a trolley and then proceeded to push me across the room. I am about six feet tall and I simply could not get used to the world from a height of two feet and to viewing events from a prone position. I resented not being in control, could not accept that I had suddenly become part of someone else's job. The trolley was in the corridor now and seemed to be accompanied by an army of marching feet. We rolled and marched into the crowded dining area, adjacent to the main reception, and I was aware briefly of the curious gaze of family groups sitting at tables. Then we were outside in the bright Nordic sunshine, I was being raised into a waiting ambulance. Iain and the younger paramedic scrambled in to the back beside me and we were off.

The motion of the ambulance soon made me feel nauseous and it was hard to concentrate on what the young man was saying. Something about measuring blood oxygen. Then a mask was over my mouth and nose. I still couldn't believe this was actually happening, but the swaying of the ambulance and the fact that I was tied down into a lying position reminded me that, however much I might like to be viewing events from the outside, I was very much involved. "I know what this is," said the paramedic. But he either did not know the English word for my illness, or else felt it was such a dread disease that he should not mention it aloud. The word "stroke" hovered in my mind but I could not absorb the thought in any meaningful way.

Iain sat quietly, still pale, and I wondered through my

tears if he was thinking back to the same events as I was – events that, almost six years before, had shocked and devastated my whole family. The feelings of deep sadness and bereavement which we'd all experienced then were now engulfing me again and as the ambulance rolled bumpily into Oslo I wept unrestrained heaving sobs that I could not bring under control.

3

Inganess Cottage

It was April 1998 and Inganess Cottage – our Orkney home – had been bruised, blinded and ravished. When we had bought it, some years previously, Inganess Cottage was empty and falling steadily into disrepair. It lacked properly functioning basic services, the roof and walls leaked generously and a chaotically tumbledown lean-to conservatory was loosely attached to one side. The house had tall chimney stacks which thrust bravely and solidly upwards in the face of regular thrashing from the Orkney gales. If you visit Kirkwall you can see it to the east of the town, spikily defined on top of a low hill. There was a fine drystane wall round the overgrown garden which, unusually for Orkney, contained a good number of mature trees, as well as an assortment of established flowering shrubs. In short, Inganess Cottage might have been described by estate agents as having "potential". The solicitor selling it had described it as a "small mansion house" – a greatly overblown description – though it had the potential to be a comfortable family home.

In April 1998, together with my colleague, Dan

Macleod, I undertook an insane cycling marathon round the colleges of the University of the Highlands and Islands. Our intention was to establish a fund for disabled students attending the University. On the day I returned, it was obvious from the moment I saw it that the old house – our home – had been subjected to a serious assault during my absence. It was early evening and I'd flown in from Inverness with my cycle in the hold of the aeroplane. While much of the ride had been uneventful, if strenuous, Dan had contracted a virus during our stay at Sabhal Mor Ostaig College on the Isle of Skye – as a result, I had completed the last leg of the trip to colleges in Oban, Perth, Elgin and Inverness on my own. The Principal of Inverness College had cycled with me from Inverness out to the airport. It was a short flight to Kirkwall and now here I was back to a home that looked as if it had been attacked by terrorists.

The large kitchen window to the front, with its view over Kirkwall, was boarded up so that the house looked like a patched stone pirate. Our car – an elderly Volvo – was parked outside. There was nothing unusual about that. In all our years at Inganess Cottage it had never once seen the inside of the small grey-rendered garage to the rear of the house. But the car was minus the glass in its rear windows and deep scratches were etched on the bodywork. Somebody had tried to patch the windows up with polythene but this had torn and now flapped forlornly in the Orkney wind. We were not a car-proud family – every vehicle we'd ever owned had been well worn before we ever turned a key in its ignition – but even for us this was a new vehicular depth.

It did not take Jo long to run through the story of what had happened.

Around 3 a.m. a few nights earlier she and the rest of the family had been sound asleep when they'd been awakened by a resounding crash – this it transpired was the kitchen window being smashed in by a boulder whose trajectory had taken it through the glass and into the kitchen where it rumbled along the floor. Similar attempts had been made on the other front windows. Shaking with fear, Jo had gone downstairs, switching lights on as she went. But whoever they were, the would-be intruders, window smashers and car vandalisers had fled, leaving behind loose boulders, broken glass, senseless destruction, a ravished family home and a terrified family.

Jo had called the police, who discovered a single large boot-print in the front garden but no other evidence of who these people might be. However, it had not taken her long to figure out that those responsible probably guessed the house would be empty – I had been speaking on Radio Orkney by telephone a few days earlier giving an update on our progress on the cycle ride, so they had probably assumed we were all out of Orkney.

What was going on here? First, for months we'd had menacing telephone calls (adult, male), now this senseless destruction. Some malevolent force in Orkney seemed to be at work, hounding us and refusing to let us be. Not for the first time, Brian Aim, builder and friend, came to the rescue, rapidly and efficiently making good all the damage to the house over the next few days. Houses can be fixed, cars can be repaired – the damage to heart and spirit lasts much longer.

We said very little to anyone, apart from one or two close friends, about the damage to our home. I hoped – forlornly, as it turned out – that I would pick up on the grapevine the names of those who had been responsible, or that someone would come and speak to me about it. Sooner or later, head teachers tend to get to hear who's alleged to have done what. Furthermore, such events are not commonplace in Orkney and most Orcadians would be appalled by such pointless destruction. But no-one said a word about it. It was as if no attack had taken place. A few weeks later, once Brian had replaced the windows and repaired the rest of the damage we tried to forget these events had ever taken place.

The Orkney summer of 1998 came and went in a blur of wind, sunshine and World Cup football. David returned to Orkney for the summer from St Andrews University, having managed to find himself a labouring job at Kirkwall harbour. Occasionally I would see him there wearing the extra-long boiler suit with which he'd been provided to fit his six-foot eight frame. When he was not working, he spent his time fishing and playing squash. He would stand for hours, waist-deep (chest-deep for anyone else) in one of the freshwater lochs or he would cast optimistically into the sea from the Churchill Barriers. The fresh mackerel and Orkney trout which he sometimes caught were a delight.

With both boys at home, and the World Cup on TV, they and their friends took up residence most evenings in our small sitting-room, with long legs, very long legs in David's case, stretched out across the carpet. Their cheers and groans (usually groans) would echo through the house. Scotland lost to Brazil in the opening match, then drew with Norway and we were finally thrashed by Morocco. Plenty of groan material there. You may wish to look away now, as they say.

David had enjoyed his first year at St Andrews University so much that his anticipation at returning in September was an almost palpable force in the house. He loved the challenge of his Marine Biology course. He loved the varied group of friends he had got to know – one of these, at least as tall as David, was following a similar course. But above all, he loved the opportunity to be himself, unencumbered by being the head teacher's son and the confines of the Orkney community. At nineteen years old, he had embarked on life. The last I saw of David that September was a rush of rucksacks and other paraphernalia being packed into our car as Jo prepared to drive him down to the ferry for Aberdeen one evening.

I wish I had savoured that moment more.

I next heard David's voice on the evening of Sunday 27 September when he telephoned home. "Hello, Dad? (a mildly antipodean, slightly querulous tonal uplift on the second word) Dad, I just phoned to wish you happy birthday – I've been in Aberdeen to watch the football. Sorry your card's a bit late, but it's on its way." I was fairly sure a girl had featured in the Aberdeen visit as well. Still, only a week late with the birthday greetings – I was impressed he'd remembered.

By the same time the following evening, 28 September 1998, David – our tall, gentle, beautiful, sport-mad, nature-loving son, our David – was dead.

"Hello, Dad?"

David had being playing in goal for his Hall of Residence team – University Hall, St Andrews. With his long arms and legs and his willingness to launch himself headlong in any direction he was a natural in this position. Over a long September evening and night, through a series of telephone calls to and from Inganess Cottage, we pieced together what had happened. At some point David had been hit in the chest by the ball, but had carried on playing. Sometime later, he had collapsed on the field, and various people had come to his aid, including a doctor who had been playing football on a neighbouring pitch. The doctor had attempted to revive him until an ambulance arrived and drove him at high speed to hospital in Dundee. On the journey the crew carried on trying to revive him. But he never recovered consciousness.

"Hello, Dad?"

As if in counterpoint to the destruction of Inganess Cottage, the Orkney community now rallied in sympathy and grief once David's death became known. Flowers filled our house. The scent of lilies hung heavy in the air. The telephone rang and rang and rang. Letters and cards arrived every day – from friends, strangers, family, colleagues, pupils.

"I don't know what to write . . ."

". . . disbelief . . ."

". . . the whole community feels deeply for you . . ."

". . . I know we have had our differences, but . . ." (from a troubled and troubling pupil)

To lose a child is unthinkable, unnatural and cruel. The love that has gone into the child, the potential for the future, the talent – all wasted. One colleague said to me: "You have lost David, you will never get him back – but no-one can take away his spirit and the memories you have of him. Keep them close."

There was a deeply moving funeral service and celebration of David's life in the austere splendour of St

Magnus Cathedral and, a few days later, a memorial service in St Salvator's Chapel, St Andrews attended by many, many of David's friends and fellow students.

"Hello, Dad?" echoed in my head for months – it echoes still – and it echoed again like a refrain as I lay in a bed in Akershus University Hospital six years later.

4

Sea Dog

I'm an old sea dog, really.

There's a picture in our home of me on a beach earlier this year –I look completely at home: a bold dog laughing in the face of the encroaching Atlantic rollers, ears flying in the wind. Oh yes, a tough old sea dog if ever there was one.

The only thing that spoils this picture is the coat I'm wearing. It's a brown woolly thing that makes me look soft and silly. I mean, how macho is that? We male whippets struggle hard enough to look big, fierce and manly without our human companions forcing us to wear such things. However, this is not the worst coat I've had. A few years ago Mistress introduced me to a horrible, blue waterproof thing that looked awful and smelled worse than a stressed cat. The first time I wore it in public a nearby dog, catching sight of me, changed his normal, friendly "Bark. Bark. Bark" into "Berk. Berk. Berk." I froze, dug my feet into the ground and refused to move another paw until Mistress took the monstrosity off me. I vowed never to wear a coat again, but Mistress has an Iron Will, so of course I've had to give in.

Anyway, back to my life as a sea dog.

Some of my earliest memories are of running along wide, empty beaches, with not another dog in sight, waves crashing on the sand, salt in the air, wind in my face and tempting morsels of rotting seagull available for comprehensive investigation placed at intervals along the beach. As a young and rather immature dog, I had enormous fun running as hard and as far as I possibly could, then thundering to a halt to investigate a salty seaside smelly, and pretending not to hear the faint calls of Master or Mistress summoning me back to their side.

The only problem with being a sea dog was that from time to time, my human companions decided to travel away from our island home. This meant actually sailing on the sea – which is quite different from simply running around beside it. The sea doesn't stay still, and while Master and Mistress luxuriated in the human part of the ship, I was left mouldering in the dark in the car-bed. The first time this happened, I didn't fully understand what was going on. When the ship left, there was much clanging and banging, which eventually gave way to a gentle throbbing and distant splashing. As time passed, however, the bowels of the ship began to heave and toss about. I could hear creaking and roaring all around me. The air reeked of oil and diesel and unhappy cows. If I may be slightly indelicate, my own bowels started to heave and toss like the ship, and I had a horrible feeling that the small bowl of food I had eaten before departure was going to make a sudden and rather unpleasant reappearance. After many trips like this, however, my bowels grew accustomed to the motion and I became a hardened sea dog, laughing in the face of the wildest seas and eagerly tucking into my pre-voyage biscuit.

For what seemed like eternity, life was one long, happy round of salt air, seaside running, roaring winds and wild heaving voyages in the car bed. I loved it. When I met other dogs, who were not fortunate enough to live by the sea, I couldn't help showing off my scent of romantic marine exoticism. There was sand between my paws, salt wind in my face and hearty fishy treats in my belly.

But, one day it all came to a sudden end.

Without so much as a by your leave, Master and Mistress took me on one of the longest car-bed journeys I have ever had, and at the end of it, there was no more sea; no salt in the air; no roaring wind; just ... silence, twittering birds and a smell of green things. I never saw home again.

Why did my human companions do this to me?

As usual, when Master and Mistress take these decisions, no explanation is offered, and as with coat-wearing, I am not consulted. I'm simply left to ponder the big questions: How is a sea dog supposed to come to terms with trees, roads and irritating inland rabbits? Where is home? Why can't humans just leave well alone? Bones and biscuits, one day they will destroy everything.

And one more question, as I roll over in my kitchen bed, trying to ignore Master's persistent call of "Walkies!" – why can't they just let sleeping dogs lie?

5

Akershus Universitetssykehus

"You have been very lucky," said the nurse called Princess. Princess was from Sierra Leone and had been asked by her colleagues to communicate with me as she was an English speaker. I was lying in bed in Ward S9 of the Akershus University Hospital on the northern edge of Oslo.

"In what way am I lucky?" I slurred resentfully through my frozen mouth.

"Because", she said "you have no bleeding into the brain. It's a blood clot. Not so difficult to treat." She pointed to a small wooden cupboard beside my bed and added, as if this was an integral part of my treatment. "This is your locker. Look after it." . . . adding, "I'll come back to test your swallowing soon." Then she was gone.

I lay on my back and thought.

After the ambulance ride, I'd been taken into a featureless white room for assessment. Injections had been given, a drip inserted into my right hand. I'd been given a brain scan and been asked a series of questions in broken English by efficient-looking men and women in white coats. Iain was a constant presence by my side.

There may well be people reading this who are old hands at being a hospital patient, to whom all of this is routine stuff. I was scared witless and at the time a virtual novice in the role of patient. It was years since I'd been at the sharp end of emergency hospital treatment – not in any serious way since the 1970s when I'd fallen off a motor bike in Cameroon, in West Africa. This was an experience which had stuck in my mind more for its humour than its pain. There, I had been treated in a room with an open glassless window, which was crammed with curious black faces observing the fine detail of a white man's naked backside being casually and very publicly injected against tetanus by a largely unsympathetic French doctor.

In this Oslo hospital, in my frozen lumpish state, there was a lot to get used to. For a start, the feeling of helplessness, the lack of any sense of being in control of what I could and couldn't do. One of the worst features of a stroke is its suddenness. If you've been used, as I was, to filling every minute of every day with something – work, leisure activities, whatever – to be reduced to lying inert for hours on end, unable to move, to read, or even sit up, quickly reduces you to despair and tears of frustration. I required the attendance of a nurse for the slightest thing – a drink of water (I passed the swallowing test), administration of pills, a bottle for peeing.

Apart from unending tearfulness, my other memory from that first day is struggling to get used to the world from a prone position, a couple of feet above the ground, instead of the usual six. I could grasp that I was not in control of the situation, that I was now part of someone else's job, a challenge for the minds and skills of professionals in whom I had to place a great deal of trust and with whom I had to co-operate if things were ever going to be any better. But to come to terms with seeing things from below – to lie prone looking up at a new world of featureless ceilings, of voices from above, of the tall able-bodied gazing down from their great height – was a new and troubling sensation.

During that first day I cautiously explored the extent of the damage. Left leg – numb and lifeless. Left arm – throbbing painlessly and lifeless, hand particularly affected. Face – left side tight and stiff, mouth slack and numb at the left hand side, chin frozen. Speech, when I tried it, effortful and drunkenly slurred. I drifted in and out of sleep for hours and was only vaguely aware of staff and other patients. There was a delicious background silence and sense of calm. Princess and her colleagues seemed to move almost noiselessly about the ward.

After travelling to the hospital, and sitting with me during the initial assessments, Iain had left to collect his car from the Rica Hotel. I think he returned later in the day to tell me he had also telephoned Jo, who had arranged to fly to Oslo that evening. At any rate, I knew she was on her way to Norway.

I spent a great deal of time in those early days at Akershus hospital asleep or lying in bed staring at the ceiling, thinking about what had happened and wondering what the prospects for recovery were. Actually, that's not true. I spent my first few days in an emotional storm, fearing the worst, angry with myself, inwardly yelling at the world, convinced that to all intents and purposes my life was over. I was 55. My life was full of interest – my own consultancy business, gardening, music, theatre, voluntary work for VSO and the Duke of Edinburgh Award Scheme – only a few days before leaving for Norway I had helped assess a group of youngsters on an Award Scheme expedition in the Grampians. Were all these things now going to come to an end? Was life, as I had known it, now over? After all, I appeared to have no functional use at all of the left hand side of my body. In the following weeks I became aware of how much worse things could have been – as well as use of arm and leg, I could have lost the power of speech or sight, I could have lost all reasoning or language skills and been unable to read, speak or understand the written word – but at that time I could not believe things could be any worse than they already were.

What I knew about stroke, could be written on the back of a very small envelope.

Jo arrived at the hospital on the Monday morning. My first concern was to reassure her that, though physically I might be largely inert, I was still in full possession of my faculties.

"I'm still the same Eric," I reassured her anxiously.

"Oh, that's disappointing," she said.

Jo has never failed to support and sustain my spirit, even when black angry moods and utter frustration drove me to despair. There must have been many days when she felt a similar despair, but she never showed it and maintained a good-humoured understanding that helped to raise my spirits and give me the emotional strength I needed.

We began to make the acquaintance of the medical staff who were looking after me. Nurses appeared, disappeared and reappeared according to their shifts. Most were women, though there were also a couple of men. They were an international group – from Finland, Sweden, Iran, Sierra Leone as well as Norway. Several spoke some English, and we got to know one or two quite well.

One nurse, an Iranian Kurd called Gelavij, described her experience of fleeing from Iran to Iraq in the late 1980s. She had been wounded in 1989 while pregnant, during one of Saddam Hussein's attacks on the Kurds, and as a result had spent several months in hospital. The baby survived. She and her family fled to Norway and had lived in Oslo for several years. She was always cheerful and constantly apologised for the quality of her English. The other nurses called her VJ as they could not get to grips with her full name. Gelavij was small, stocky and dark-haired and regularly had the responsibility of helping me to shower. As I could not stand, the procedure was that she would wheel me along to the shower room, help me to strip and transfer to a shower chair, usually with the help of a colleague, and then turn the powerful shower hose on me. Using my good hand I would try to make the best of shampooing, soaping up and shaving. Then she would rinse me off, dry me and wheel me back to my room. I felt like a helpless infant.

On one occasion she had to leave me alone in the shower room. She was gone for less than a minute but in that short time I managed to drop a piece of soap and, in leaning over for it, over-balanced from my shower chair, fell leadenly to the floor and banged my head on the toilet pan. My howl of shock brought her hurrying back, along with two other nurses who hauled me back into the shower chair. Gelavij was inconsolable ... "that this should happen to my patient" ... "I shouldn't have left you." On one level it was comic, I was writhing around completely naked like a beached fish on the shower room floor, but to me, it was not the fall itself but the powerlessness of scrabbling about, unable to raise myself from the shower-room floor, that seemed to underline the humiliation and wholly dependent state in which I now existed. I dealt with it in the only way I seemed capable of articulating anything – by bursting into tears.

The consultant responsible for monitoring my treatment was an extremely caring man who spoke excellent English. He had me wheeled along to his office from time to time, and would check on my progress as well as explaining calmly more about the type of stroke I'd suffered – a lacunar stroke, which he said was caused by a tiny gap or blockage in a fine artery somewhere in the brain. He also said they had been unable to pinpoint the clot in the MRI scan that I'd had on first admission to the hospital. He did various checks on my carotid arteries and legs to ensure no other clots were lurking. It seemed to me absolutely incredible that such a tiny pinhead of blood could result in such total destruction, and that such a small area of the brain was responsible for so many activities – in my case the absence of my left arm and leg would mean I could no longer do such much-loved activities as walking the dog, climbing hills, gardening and playing the violin, not to mention such mundane tasks as tying shoe-laces or wiping my backside. I kept thinking of the things I couldn't – wouldn't ever again – do and as these thoughts welled up so did the tears of frustration, regret and self-pity.

On one visit the consultant said, "You have youth on your side."

This is not something that is often said to a 55-year old man, so my initial reaction was to preen myself mentally – obviously I couldn't physically preen myself – and I sat more upright in my wheelchair.

"What do you mean?" I said

"The younger you are the more elastic your brain is. You can relearn how to do things."

This joined the new store of facts I was accumulating about stroke.

A couple of days after my arrival in the hospital, I was moved from the main ward to a smaller room, which housed two of us. My room-mate was an eighty-six year old man, Trygve Blomset, who spoke no English, and who spent much of the time with his bed surrounded by the long, white hospital curtains. We would smile at one another on those occasions when the curtains were not drawn. At least once a day, a nurse would arrive, whisk the curtains closed around his bed and administer some kind of treatment which reduced the normally cheerful old man to sobbing howls of pain.

My bed was close to the window and I gradually grew familiar with the sounds of the Oslo suburb outside – the murmuring rhythms of traffic, the occasional sound of horns or brakes and very close at hand the rumbles and clatters from an enormous building site where the foundations of an entirely new hospital were being built. From time to time, a whistle or horn would sound and a few moments later there would be a loud blast and the whole room would shake as rock was blown apart to clear the way for building work. It seemed surprising to me that a new hospital was being built when the one I was currently housed in seemed more than adequate. Not only did it appear solidly constructed, it was spotlessly clean and kept so by an army of quietly efficient cleaning staff. All hospital staff dressed in a plain white uniform – from consultants to cleaners – and this uniform, we learned, was kept in the hospital as well as being laundered and cleaned there. Individual members of staff were identified by a badge, pinned to their chest which stated their name and the title of the post they held.

From early on in my stay at the Akershus Universitetssykehus I was seen by a couple of physiotherapists – one a Lebanese woman, small, swarthy, chatty and an excellent English speaker conducted the first examination of my flaccid body. I was seated on a firm bed, she removed my t-shirt, leaving me in my shorts, and then moved aside to let me see myself in a large mirror at the opposite side of the room. I was horrified by what I saw. I was looking at someone only vaguely resembling the person I had been. My mouth had a severe downward twist to the left. My left shoulder sloped oddly and, but for her lightly restraining hand, I would have keeled over to the left. But, above all, I was staring at the image of someone old, feeble and wholly unlike the man who'd flown in to Bergen a few days earlier.

The physiotherapist performed a thorough examination of my sagging left-hand side muscles and tested my levels of sensation at various points. She then asked me to use my left side to perform various activities, none of which I could manage. The attempt to perform any of these activities – raising my arm, moving my fingers, straightening my leg, standing up – required a Herculean effort and made me simply want to collapse weakly into her arms and cry. Over the next couple of days I also met her Norwegian colleague : a tall, slim, rather stern lady about my own age. Her name badge told me she was Gunhilde Sexe and she informed me that her husband was a senior officer in the Norwegian army. I could well believe it. On our first acquaintance she dragged me out of my wheelchair and frogmarched me after a fashion along the corridor from my ward to the physiotherapy room. She achieved this by grasping my shoulders from behind and kicking the back of my left knee each time I took a step. Jo followed pushing the empty wheelchair that went everywhere with me. I felt like a drunk being frogmarched home after a night out. But I am now convinced that if I'd had more of this rough but well-intentioned treatment persistently throughout my rehabilitation in Scotland, I would have made faster progress. However, in those early days even the short daily spells of physiotherapy exhausted me so completely that I slept for hours afterwards.

In general the staff in the Oslo hospital had a much more hands-on approach to their patients than I was later to experience from most of their British colleagues. This was partly out of necessity as they did not have the plethora of hoists and lifts which I later encountered in Scotland. Day after day a nurse, invariably smaller and slighter than myself, would haul me between bed and wheelchair. Gelavij, for example, despite her small size, was perfectly capable of heaving me out of my wheelchair and manoeuvring me heavily on to my bed. Doubtless a British health and safety person observing this procedure would have demanded that the hospital authorities provide a proper hoist forthwith to protect the welfare of nurse and patient. Perhaps they would have been right to do so, but the net result of all this manhandling was a feeling of being wanted and cared for, of being helped. There was a physical communication there which said, "We want to help. We know it's difficult for you. But we're interested and involved in this business of conquering your stroke." Is there a health and safety measure for the *absence* of communication, the *absence* of care, the *absence* of interest?

For the first day or two, I ate very little. But gradually I felt able to face more food. Meals were brought to the room that Trygve and I shared. The food was excellent.

Although there was no choice and the portions were small, it was always healthy – fruit, vegetables, a small portion of fish, fruit drinks, and an endless supply of water. After the first few days, Jo was able to wheel me along to the small patients' lounge and sometimes I would eat my meal at a table placed at one end of this room. Here, I began to master the art of eating with one hand, clumsily cutting things up with a knife held in my right hand, frequently spilling drinks and tired after sitting upright for only a short time in the wheelchair.

A few days after I was moved into the room with Trygve, a parcel arrived for me from the UK. Jo opened it for me. It contained a letter, a small portable cassette player and some tapes. These had been sent by good friends in Aberdeenshire. They were a godsend. Most of the tapes were BBC recordings of the radio programme "I'm Sorry I haven't a Clue" – I listened for hours to the tapes, with the portable earphones planted one in each ear, while Trygve or a nurse would gaze in surprise at my good right shoulder heaving with laughter. Perhaps the future might be brighter after all. In any case, I was going to work on my recovery, wasn't I?

I knew that I could not stay indefinitely in the hospital. I wanted to return home, and, of course, Jo could not continue to stay on in the hotel for much longer either – she had taken over the room I'd vacated. I had an annual travel insurance policy, and Iain volunteered to contact the insurance company to try to make arrangements for my return to Scotland. This proved a challenge. Initially, the company suggested that I should get a taxi to Oslo airport, jump on a scheduled flight to Heathrow, take a second flight from there to Aberdeen, then check myself in to hospital. Iain attempted to explain the impossibility of this, but the company were clearly not prepared to be persuaded by the arguments of a 22-year old boy. There was also a query from them about why Jo needed to be there at all. After several days of telephone calls, faxes, tears from me (again), anger and tears from Jo, then finally an angry telephone call to the insurance company from the normally mild-mannered hospital consultant, they eventually agreed to provide an ambulance plane that would fly both Jo and myself from Oslo to Aberdeen.

Once this had been agreed we awaited the receipt of a fax by the hospital to confirm dates and times. Unbelievably, there was then a quibble from the insurance company about how I was to get to Oslo airport and who was to pay for the ambulance. I do not know to this day how this was finally resolved – though all the goodwill and caring appeared to be on the Norwegian side.

On 29 July 2004 – 11 days after I had first been wheeled into Akershus Universitetssykehus – I was wheeled out again and tied into a stretcher in one of the smallest ambulances I had ever seen. Jo squeezed in beside me and we set off for the airport. We had to be driven to a very far corner of the airport (I gathered), where the ambulance drew up. The rear doors of the ambulance opened. Through them I could see a small aircraft from which emerged a rump – or at least, a rump with a nurse's uniform pasted around about it. She squeezed herself through the aircraft's door, bumped heavily down the aircraft's two or three steps and stood four-square beside the ambulance.

I raised my head slightly and looked at her through the rear doors of the ambulance.

"Ow, can't he walk then? We don't have a stretcher," she said, ignoring me and speaking over my head to my wife.

I was about to re-enter the real world.

6

Small Humans

I am trying to shut out the world.

When I want to do this I burrow under a comfortable, dark blue blanket with a pattern of white paw prints all over it which lies in my kitchen bed. In the last few days I have spent rather a lot of time under it – in fact, I am under it right now, so please excuse me if my words seem a bit mumbled.

A wise dog once told me that there are three ages of dog:

1. the age of puppyhood
2. the middle-age, and
3. the age of "aren't you looking well".

I fear I may now have entered the third of those ages, because not only do I want to keep a low profile, but I feel very, very tired. Let me explain.

Normally, I feel quite young when I first wake up. Most mornings, before the day properly begins, I lie in bed stretching my legs, yawning, shaking my tail and scratching – basically checking that everything is functioning as it should – and at that stage I often think to myself "Hamish, you're feeling fine. You look pretty fine. The day is young. Life is good. Look out cats and rabbits. Let's go." This thought is then followed by a joyous leap out of bed.

But today I seem to have entered the third age and I am keeping a low profile because a tornado has struck our normally peaceful home – Rachel and her children have come to stay with us.

Rachel is the eldest child of Master and Mistress and years ago she used to accompany me on walks. Together we would wander down country paths, along beaches, through forests. It was companionable and pleasant. Nowadays, however, Rachel is mistress to two small children who accompany her everywhere. Both are very small, but one is slightly taller than the other. He is tall enough to look me straight in the eye, but, despite this, he finds me scary and screams if I go near him. I ask you – me scary? I don't think so. Master's ruffled early morning appearance – now that's scary. Mistress exercising her fearsome Iron Will – that's scary. But me, Hamish, gentle silver whippet with a long white stripe down my face and mournful brown eyes – I don't think I'm scary at all.

Anyway, whatever confidence the slightly larger child lacks in the presence of a dog, the smaller child more than makes up for in boldness in the presence of anything and everything. He appears to wear a great deal of padding between his plump little legs. As he can barely walk, he stomps around waving his little arms and squawking at the top of his voice like a demented duck. Occasionally, he falls with a thud to the floor on the thick padding that surrounds his bottom. He has a nose moister than that of any dog I've known. He enjoys nothing more than patting me inappropriately with his small fists. By "inappropriately" I am delicately hinting at the fact that he does not know one end of a dog from the other. Fortunately, I am patient as well as handsome, so I simply adopt a pained expression and pretend nothing unusual has happened.

Master tells me that one day both of these children will grow up and be like most other humans – i.e. reliable but unexciting (much like Master himself). In the meantime, they are unpredictable. For example, both of them rain huge quantities of food on to the floor when they are eating at table. This I like. I sit staring up at them with my jaws gaping in the hope that morsels will come my way. However, if, at some later point, I happen upon one of them holding a small biscuit and try to share it with him, the child involved will start to yell and scream and Mistress will send me to a distant corner of the house in disgrace – or worse still, I'll be sent outside to lie in the car bed, far removed from any eating opportunities.

Then again, the children appear to own a huge

collection of colourful toys, some of which squeak and rattle in quite an exciting way. They bash, squeak, rattle and throw these toys all day long. I can relate to this, but the moment I try to join in their game by doing the same thing, you can be sure that one of them will howl like a distressed bloodhound, and I'll be banished to the outer darkness.

So, this morning I have decided to keep a low profile, partly so that I can avoid being punished for bad behaviour, and partly so that I can recover from a night of broken sleep caused by the smaller child screaming endlessly for his mistress. Also, I have a belief that if I just lie here, life's tornadoes will eventually blow themselves out. There will come a time when I can creep out from under the dark blue blanket with white paw prints all over it. The tornado will have passed. There will be no more yelling and screaming. No more inappropriate patting. No more spells of disgrace in the car bed.

And I can just get on with enjoying the third age of dog.

7

Aberdeen

Leaving Norway and travelling back to Aberdeen had been a bit like coming to the end of a holiday. The stay in Akershus hospital had had a foreign, holiday-time, dream-like quality to it despite its unpleasant medical aspects. Rest and recuperation were now over. It was time now to get back to the routine of work and normality. Except, of course, for me there would be no work. And no normality.

The plane journey was a kind of transition back to reality.

Lying inside the ambulance plane was rather like being in a coffin. I was laid out and tied on to a flat bed in the centre of the passenger compartment. My head was towards the front of the plane. Jo sat on a seat just behind my head. The nurse was seated just beyond my feet. Somewhere ahead, the pilot was (presumably) firmly set on his course for Aberdeen. A couple of feet above me, were the red curtain-like pleats of the material that shrouded the interior of the plane. The engine noise drilled into my head with an endless deafening rhythm.

We had levelled out and were suspended at 10,000 feet above ragged Norwegian mountains and fjords. I couldn't see them, of course, but somehow that was all the more terrifying – enclosed space, small plane, unrelenting noise and vibration, a thin layer of metal and miles of silent empty air between us and an unforgiving rocky death. I didn't want Jo to see my fear – she doesn't particularly enjoy flying and normally closes her eyes and grips her armrest with tight white knuckles during take-off and landing.

After we had been going some time, I needed to pee. I always needed to pee these days. In hospital the nurses had always discreetly left a supply of plastic bottles beside my bed. Presumably, a supply of these was available on the plane.

"I need to use the ..."

The nurse immediately began guddling around in a bag and produced a plastic bottle while Jo helped to undo my zip.

I used to have a teaching colleague many years ago who had carried his RAF days with him into the staffroom (and classroom, too, presumably). He had a red face and a thatch of reddish hair. His recollections were often difficult to believe. "There I was, upside down, nothing on the clock but the maker's name ..." he'd say and then launch into some far-fetched exploit alleged to have happened in 1943 or whenever, his face becoming redder and redder with excitement. Well, here I was, lying on my back, nothing in my tank, struggling to pee into a plastic bottle, no-one in the plane but the pilot, the woman I loved and a fat nurse, with me scared beyond measure of falling into an unseen Norwegian fjord thousands of feet below.

It was a relief when, after a long, long time, we felt the plane begin to descend. There was a brief moment when I had a vision of my head banging on to the airport tarmac, but then we were down and the wheels were rolling along with a rubbery hum to our allotted parking place in a distant corner of the airport, where crocks like me would not be seen by the fare-paying public.

Silence. Then a hiatus of some minutes, during which the unseen pilot flicked switches and folded up a map. An ambulance eventually drove up. The reverse of the procedures at Oslo was enacted, the fat nurse said her goodbyes and we were bumping towards Aberdeen Royal Infirmary.

Akershus Hospital had been striking for its sense of calm, despite the adjacent enormous building site. Ward 11 of Aberdeen Royal Infirmary was a raucous cacophony of noise. It was Saturday evening when I was wheeled in on a trolley. Near my bed a large television set flickered garishly and trashily, the volume turned to maximum. To one side I was aware of a rank of inert, prone elderly patients. In a room attached to the end of the ward I could hear the incessant, desperate shout of a woman calling "Nurse! Nurse! Nurse!" In another corner of the ward a gaggle of nursing staff shouted, belched, swore and gossiped at the top of their voices. They appeared to be oblivious to the noisy, desolate, hellish scene around them, seeking only to shout above it.

I wanted to run. Failing that (and obviously I did), I wanted to be back in the soothing calm of Ward S9 Akershus. Communication might sometimes have been a problem, but at least there was a general background of peace and quiet. Above all, the staff there did not shout in the presence of patients and there was no television set in the ward. During my stay in this ward, it seemed to me that no-one had trained the staff to look hard at how the hospital experience might appear from a patient's point of view. A few individuals did try to make this leap of imagination and they stood out like gold nuggets in a shale pile, but on the whole, for the patient who was feeling tired and unwell (and surely that must be the majority), Ward 11 did not seem to be the place to find inner calm.

On my first full, working day in Aberdeen Royal, I was wheeled into the physiotherapy department to be assessed briefly by a harassed physiotherapist. Later in the day I was told by a young doctor that the ward I was in was really intended for ill people, and that, since I didn't fall into that category (I assumed he was joking) as soon as a bed became available I would be moved to the Stroke Rehabilitation Unit at Woodend Hospital, a short distance away. No-one could tell me how long I would have to wait for this but many described the Woodend Unit as a kind of stroke survivor's heaven ("they do wonderful things there" was a typical comment), providing first class, frequent, intensive physiotherapy and general care. I assumed this would mean resuming the daily physiotherapy I had enjoyed in Norway and looked forward eagerly to the transfer there. It was now two weeks since my stroke, and I knew from the Norwegian physiotherapists that it was important to get active as soon as possible to promote recovery. I still had a vague and somewhat naïve view of what the word "rehabilitation" meant in the context of Woodend Hospital's "Unit". "Woodend" had a pleasantly sylvan ring to it. In my more upbeat moments, I pictured in my mind miserable paralysed patients being wheeled in there one day on a stretcher and then on another day a few weeks later striding happily and confidently out, throwing away all sticks and walking aids, having been put through an intensive programme of physical restoration.

I had this view partly because I still regarded the consequences of the stroke as purely physical – in my case, an arm and a leg, and to some extent a mouth, face and voice, would have to be put right with a series of tedious but necessary exercises. After all, you get ill, you go to hospital, they hurt you for your own good, you get cured, you leave, you resume your life. Isn't that how it works?

Not with stroke.

Stroke is both instant and insidious, and every stroke is different. In simple terms, the initial "insult" – in my case a blood clot – starves part of the brain of oxygen. If the oxygen supply is not restored within a short time, the brain cells in that locality die, and so the parts of your body controlled by those cells cease to function. The body's rather miraculous repair process gradually allows other parts of the brain to take over the functions of the dead cells (at least that's the theory), hence recovery, which may be over days, weeks, months, years. No medical person can honestly put a time limit on how long any individual will take to recover – or indeed how fully they will recover. Awkward for the patient. Awkward for the medical staff. Awkward for the bean counters who control the system. With our money, our beans.

And there's more.

The body is not like a computer where you can replace a faulty circuit with a new one. The body feels. The body is alive with present perceptions, past memories and future hopes. The body is human, and therefore unpredictable. So far as I could see, the medical "experts" in Aberdeen seemed to be treating my body more like a machine than a human being with a past, a present medical condition and – hopefully – a future. No one in Aberdeen spent time with me answering the huge pressing questions that constantly occupied my mind.

As I lay rotting in Ward 11, listening to the background symphony of elderly groans and farting, the harsh shouting of the nurses, and the braying of day-time television, I was gradually becoming more and more aware of the insidious effects of the stroke I'd suffered. During waking hours, I marshalled them in my mind, patrolled them in front of me one by one.

Concentration – gone. I could read words, but couldn't concentrate long enough to read more than a couple of sentences. In any case, holding a book was difficult; holding a newspaper, impossible. Worst of all, I couldn't concentrate on more than one thing at a time. No change there, Jo would say. But now it was serious. Friends had begun to visit me and I found that I couldn't focus properly on what they were saying if there was another visitor talking at the next bed, or if a nurse was speaking at the other end of the ward, or if the television was switched on (it always was).

Speech – improving, but still hard work to form the words and string them together.

Emotions – in turmoil, and out of control. I could weep for Britain. Equally, if someone made a mildly funny remark, I could not contain my bursts of laughter. Surely it could only be a matter of time before I laughed at something tragic and lost a friend forever.

Exhaustion – constant and bone-sapping. The daily routine of showering and toileting supported by wheelchair and nurse left me weak and ready to sleep. I spent the whole day in bed. I slept for hours every day. I wakened every morning as if from deep unconsciousness.

Underlying all of these side-effects, a deeper nagging question – was I really the same Eric, as I had so confidently claimed to be when Jo first came to see me in Norway. I know that other stroke survivors have felt the same – are the pre-stroke person and the post-stroke person one and the same personality? How could I know for sure?

And the biggest questions of all – was life over as I'd known it up till now? Would I recover? Would I recover completely, partially or not at all? How could I help my recovery? None of the medical staff I spoke to in Ward 11 seemed willing or able to tackle these huge questions with me.

I hoped things would be better at Woodend.

Eventually, the day came when I was wheeled from the psychological torture of Ward 11 to a waiting ambulance and from there through the city to Woodend Hospital. One thing I had established about Woodend was that it was on the correct side of Aberdeen for travel from Bogarn – Jo's journey to visit me would be shorter, if only by a couple of miles. Another way of looking at it – the only positive way of looking at it – was that by going to Woodend I was also going a couple of miles nearer home.

Jo was waiting when I was wheeled on my stretcher into the Woodend Stroke Unit. I had a brief glimpse of a small flat-roofed building as I was pushed through the automatic doors. But it was not so much the physical surroundings that I noticed, as the other patients. I was wheeled into a ward with five other men in it, all lying in their beds in various states of stillness and awareness. All of them seemed to be old men, but then I thought of my own appearance in the mirror back in Oslo: in the world's eyes I was an old man now as well. All of us had something in common – we'd survived a stroke, and were now learning to deal with the consequences.

One man, bearded, with cassette earpieces in his ears, appeared marginally more alert than the others and raised a hand as I was wheeled past. Then curtains were drawn around me – a sure sign of some medical attention heading my way.

8

Hissing Kitten

Those of you who know Master well will realise that he is far from being a genius. However, I sometimes wonder if what he lacks in mental sharpness he makes up for in his understanding of a dog's mind. This thought was provoked some time ago by watching a *cat*, of all things. You will have gathered from some of my previous ramblings that normally I regard cats with distaste.

Here are five of the reasons:

1. They can't bark.
2. If they wag their tails, it doesn't necessarily mean they are happy.
3. They hiss and spit when I go near them.
4. They have needle-sharp claws.
5. They have no sense of humour.

When I was a young dog, those beliefs were based on theory and prejudice – I had no real experience of living with cats. Then, one day, a few years ago, Mistress thought she would introduce a kitten into our perfectly happy home. I first became aware of the creature one afternoon when I was lying in one of my favourite sunny spots in a post-lunch stupor.

I will say this for Mistress – she didn't just thrust this ghastly little monster into my face and expect me to relate to it. No, she placed the hissing, twitching grey and white fur ball in the next door room. It was separated from me by a glass door. I suppose her thinking was that I would gradually get used to this intruder, accept its presence and therefore resist my basic instinct – which was to grab the horrid little moggy by its neck, shake it around a bit, then toss it in the air before deciding whether I should eat it for lunch or dinner. Anyway, I spent some time glaring at it through the glass door while it screamed and spat at me from the other side like a demented steam engine. Welcome to our happy home? I think not, you screeching, hissing little pussy cat!

I would not like you to think from the above that I am a vicious or violent dog. On the contrary, we whippets, as Master will assure you, are laid-back, gentle, easy-going creatures. It's just that there is a cat-shaped image in my brain which fills me with a desire to chase, shake and destroy (there is another rabbit-shaped image close by). All other images in my brain are completely harmless and relate mainly to biscuits and bones.

But, back to the hissing kitten. Over the next few

weeks I would growl every time she came near (the kitten was a she-cat) – she in turn would hiss, stretch her claws and arch her back. I spent some time observing the kitten's response to my various actions. If I went to eat from my bowl, up she would pop and try to pinch some of my favourite titbits. She was a greedy little monster. If I lay down to give myself some grooming, she would do the same, some distance away. Her worst habit was jumping on to Mistress's lap. I'm not allowed to do that, and on those few occasions where I have attempted to jump up, Mistress has expressed her disapproval very clearly. Master would allow me on to his lap, but Mistress does not rate his skills of dog discipline very highly. I know this because I've heard her lecturing him about it. Mistress not only allowed puss on to her lap, she stroked and petted her as well. I was horrified and I couldn't understand why Mistress didn't feel fear of the cat's claws, which puss had already used a couple of times to box me when I went too close. But worse even than those claws, I discovered to my horror that my usual attack strategy – speed – was not enough to terrify puss.

We whippets are pretty sharp movers, but I quickly learned that if I chased the kitten it could dive into the smallest of hidey holes where I simply couldn't follow. On one memorable occasion, this left me colliding painfully and clumsily with a stone wall. I was just grateful that no-one was around to witness the scrambled mess of legs and tail that I became as I skidded into that wall side-on when I tried to compensate for pussy cat's last minute dive to the left. To overcome my injured feelings and regain some dignity, I barked loudly and repeatedly at the small shrub into which puss had dived. This alerted Mistress to the fact that all was not well. You would have expected Mistress of all people to realise that this commotion had been caused by the kitten, but no, no, no! I, Hamish, was blamed for making too much noise: "Stop that silly barking at once," said Mistress, exercising her Iron Will. I slunk away, suitably chastened. That's something else we whippets are good at – slinking. Quite clearly, puss was trouble and if we didn't sort out some way of rubbing along together, one of us would have to slink away for good.

One day, however, the scales fell from my eyes, the bones fell from my plate, the treats slid from the table – I had a blinding flash, a revelation. I suddenly realised that pussy cats may, just may, have some things to teach a whippet. Well, one thing at least. It was a sunny spring day and there was a strong whiff of rabbit in the air. Puss had obviously caught this whiff as well. This interest in rabbits and a desire to tear them limb from limb was the one thing that seemed to unite us. My technique for catching rabbits is simple – I smell them, I see them, I run after them at top speed and if I'm lucky I catch them. It doesn't always work, of course, but it's simple and direct, and, apart from a short burst of running, it doesn't take much effort. It's a mindless, whippety activity.

Puss's approach was different. On that particular morning I watched from a distance as she pressed herself into the ground and then in slow controlled bursts gradually slunk – "slunk" is the only suitable word – nearer and nearer to the rabbit. The rabbit, being a rabbit, was nibbling grass and looking stupidly and nervously around from time to time. It didn't notice her remorseless approach. I was fascinated and absorbed. I couldn't help myself. "Go, pussy, go!" I whispered inwardly to my rabbit-addled brain, as she crept nearer the gormless bunny. "Go, pussy!" I almost barked out loud. By now puss was only a couple of leaps away, and still the rabbit hadn't seen her. She was poised to pounce and sink teeth and claws into bunny's neck, when the rabbit spotted her and ran like a . . . well, like a whippet, into some nearby trees. Puss did not give chase, but looked round and caught sight of me. "Tough luck, puss," I barked, and ambled back to my kitchen food bowl. But just for a moment a bond had been formed between us, and what is more, puss had shown me a whole new technique of sneaking up on rabbits which I couldn't wait to try out for myself.

From that day on, puss and I weren't friends exactly, but we tolerated each other. She kept her claws to herself, and I no longer harboured any thoughts of chasing and eating her. The evening after puss had shown me this new rabbit stalking method, Master said a strange thing. He turned to Mistress over their rather sweet-smelling supper and said to her, "There's more than one way to skin a rabbit." Had Master been watching puss as well? Is Master wiser than he looks?

As I said before, what he lacks in mental sharpness, he possibly makes up for in understanding the workings of a dog's mind.

9

Woodend

Life at the stroke unit at Woodend Hospital quickly developed into a dull, predictable daily round. I felt I was becalmed in a backwater, that the main current of life was roaring along somewhere over there through the trees and now passing me by.

Each day began in the same way. At about 7 a.m. the nursing night shift would hand over to their day time colleagues. The first sounds we inmates heard in the morning was of their chat over tea – raucous, sometimes filthy, laughter would mingle with more serious professional exchanges about the condition of this patient or that – never loud enough to be heard distinctly, but loud enough for occasional snippets to leak out.

From 7.30 a.m. onwards the process of morning bathing, showering and washing of the inmates began. In my early days in Woodend, this process was a repetition of the procedures I'd grown used to in Oslo and Aberdeen – a thorough hosing down in a special shower chair by a nurse. Over the weeks, however, I was gradually allowed more and more control over my own ablutions, and with that increased control came a slightly stronger sense of personal dignity and pride.

The stroke unit housed about twenty male and female patients – some had been in residence there for many, many months. There appeared to be two consultants attached to the unit, each with his own group of patients. The building consisted of a long corridor, off which extended three small wards with half a dozen beds in each. Each ward had one toilet and wash hand basin. There were two or three single rooms each with individual toilets and wash hand basin. In addition there was a large patients' lounge and dining room, and at the very far end there was a physiotherapy room and a small staff office. The air was hot and stagnant. Most patients were in their seventies, eighties or nineties, several were unable to speak and most were physically disabled to a greater or lesser degree. The whole place had the funereal atmosphere of a home for old people.

At a central point in the corridor, just opposite the patients' lounge was a large noticeboard on which the timetable of patient "activities" was displayed. This indicated the times at which each patient would be seen by occupational therapists and by physiotherapists. I was horrified to discover that I would usually be seen by the physiotherapists only twice a week for half-hour sessions – far less than had been the case in Oslo. Above all else, I wanted to be mobile again and I was frustrated that there would not be more opportunity to try to reactivate my rapidly wasting and stiffening muscles. I complained early on to the consultant about this. He said it came down to finance (only two physiotherapists were allocated to the unit) and that I should complain formally to the health board. I felt weak, vulnerable and frustrated and had no idea how to do this. I needed an advocate with a good knowledge of the health system to take on this challenge.

Outside brief sessions with the physiotherapists and the occupational therapists, patients lay on their beds, chatted (where they could) or met with visitors in the patients' lounge or in the wards. A television set blared constantly in each ward and more and more I found this constant background noise to be unbearable. It is a common feature of stroke, that concentration is badly affected. I quickly found that any noise or background activity was an impossible distraction – the constantly braying television was the worst of all, making it impossible to concentrate on talking to other patients or visitors, to read or even to sleep.

Jo was a daily presence – usually staying from late morning until early evening. Sometimes she would wheel me to the hospital café; occasionally, while the weather was still warm, we'd sit in a small garden adjacent to the stroke unit. Friends visited frequently and provided a vital link to a richer life.

I was still reliant on someone pushing me around in

a wheelchair. But gradually the physiotherapists taught me to transfer from bed to chair, and chair to bed. They eventually told me to practise standing for ten to fifteen minutes each day, and a support frame was made available in case I felt dizzy or tired whilst standing up. Trying not to hold on to this frame, I would stand for as long as possible in the evening. Occasionally I would raise my right arm and exchange Nazi-style salutes with one of the men in a nearby bed.

One day in early September, I was measured for a leg splint. This, I was told, would enable me to bear weight properly on my left leg and possibly allow me to walk around independently. While this was to some extent welcome news, I did not care for the thought that this splint would become a lifelong feature, and said as much to the nursing staff and physiotherapists. "Will I have to wear this for the rest of my life?" I asked. At this there was much uttering of noncommittal sounds and shrugging of shoulders.

A week or so later the splint arrived and gradually I was allowed to hobble short distances – two or three steps initially – and at once became aware of how long a road I still had to travel before I could hope to be free of the wheelchair and dependence on other people for getting around.

The longer I stayed in Woodend, the more I became aware of the way our health service works. It is a service of specialisms. Each medical professional has his or her own jealously guarded area of professional expertise. The splint, for example, was manufactured by the orthotics department, whose silent operatives seemed to be under instruction to carry out their measuring and fitting without any undue communication with the patient they were treating.

To be fair to the staff in Woodend, they were mostly pleasant and caring and it was obvious in the stroke unit that they tried hard to work as a team. They had regular team meetings involving all medical staff and other health professionals. However, the whole system as far as quality of patient care was concerned came down to the actions of a few enthusiastic, sensitive staff who instinctively viewed things from a patient perspective. What is the point of lots of team meetings, targets and agreed approaches if the two nurses escorting a wheelchair-bound patient to the toilet talk loudly over his head about their personal lives or the latest pay grade dispute within the NHS? All the highest flown ambitions and improvement plans count for nothing if the toilets are filthy or the showers uncleaned.

I often looked around the stroke unit with its lines of inert patients, limited equipment and insufficient staffing and asked myself if this is the best we can do as a wealthy, civilised country for stroke survivors, particularly younger stroke survivors – and at 55 I counted myself as a relatively young stroke survivor.

Surely it made economic sense that people of working age should receive sufficient treatment so that they could, where possible, leave hospital as independent, tax-paying contributors to society.

During one gruelling session the young physiotherapist grinding her elbow into my left buttock said through her panting breath that she had really – gasp – enjoyed a recent in-service training course.

"What did they tell you?" I gasped back at her. "Listen to your patient?"

"Yes. That was exactly" – gasp – "the message. How did you know?"

There were still aspects of my stroke I did not understand. Why did I have a stroke in the first place? How much recovery could I expect? How long would it all take? So far, I had only vague answers to these questions – but I was beginning to understand more, through talking to staff at Woodend and later, after leaving hospital, through reading about stroke and researching medical and academic papers on the internet.

Why did I have a stroke? Prior to 18 July 2004, I had been reasonably fit and active – walking, cycling and gardening regularly. I had been taking medication for high blood pressure, and this appeared to be well under control at the time. Jo and I grew and ate vast quantities of fruit and vegetables in our well-tended plot of ground. Neither of us smoked. Neither of us drank excessively. No obvious causes there, then. However, throughout the nineties I had suffered severe migraines, sometimes for days on end. If you enter "migraine" and "stroke" into a search engine, you quickly discover that a link between migraine and stroke has been suspected for years but (at the time of writing) is not definitively proven. But when you add to this, in my case, several unpleasant spells of tinnitus, a stressful job and David's sudden death, other factors begin to suggest themselves.

I began to realise these connections only because, too late, I had time to think about them in the long, grindingly dull routine of Woodend Hospital. Hindsight, as they say, is wonderful. Should these risk factors for stroke have occurred to my GP when I presented myself to him for inspection at regular intervals? Should I myself have been more alert to them?

Then again, how much recovery could I expect? How long would it all take? The questions no doctor will answer. Every stroke is different – this was a mantra recited by all medical staff I encountered. I was learning that I had been comparatively lucky, as Princess had told me. On the debit side, my left arm was still virtually useless, and my left shoulder painful – "subluxed", said the physios, and applied various strappings to it to keep it in a good position. My left leg was slowly improving and there was a possibility I would walk again, albeit imperfectly and slowly, and perhaps only with the wretched splint. Speech was problematic and exhausting because of facial weakness. Emotions were still in turmoil.

On the credit side, unlike some of my fellow Woodend inmates, I could at least speak. I could think and reason (when the television was switched off). I was "reading" books again by listening to them on CD. It was possible I might return to work one day. I might even drive a car. I was continent. I had a loving wife and family.

I was alive.

10

Spring

Spring has sprung. The grass is a juicy green. There's a whiff of daffodils and young rabbit in the air. Flowers and green shoots are everywhere. It's the time of year to make a handsome silver brindle whippet with a white stripe down his nose leap for joy, joy, joy.

But I fear spring is also a time for Em o' Tee … Let me explain.

We whippets are sight hounds. Give me a distant glimpse of a cat and I'm your dog – I'll chase and run and run and run till that cat is done for. I'm a scent hound, too. Just a gentle whiff of rabbit and my nose is up and I'm off speeding towards it with the prospect of a tasty meal making my heart sing. But a hearing hound? No, I'm not so hot on hearing – which is sometimes an advantage. For example, if I'm tearing after a rabbit, the last thing I want is to hear Mistress shouting, "Come back here, Hamish!"… so I pretend not to hear it, and if I haven't heard the words, how can I obey them? However, often I genuinely don't hear, or, rather as it turns out, often I *mis*-hear.

So it was with Em o' Tee.

"Time for Em o' Tee," I was sure I'd heard Mistress say one sunny spring morning a few years ago, when I was still a young, rather naïve dog.

At first, in my innocence, I assumed Em must be an Irish girl known to Master. It's not uncommon for Master to say things to Mistress such as "Many a woman would give her right arm to be with me on this lovely sunny day." I've never really understood such comments, but these remarks have led me to believe that there are hosts of one-armed women out there who would like to usurp Mistress' position as Master's loyal companion. I imagined Em o' Tee must be one of those women. The feeling was strengthened later that same fine spring day when I thought I heard Master saying to Mistress, "Em o' Tee today." He followed up this remark with a leer in my direction. I winked back in some embarrassment. Anyway, the upshot of this comment was that we – Master, Mistress and I – jumped into the car bed and drove off – to see Em, I assumed. I am privileged to have my own personal door into the car bed, and for a while, as we rolled along, I stood gazing out at the fresh spring sunshine, noting with some frustration a number of neighbourhood cats slinking about, taking the air, with not a dog in sight to keep them in their place.

After a short sleep, I wakened with a start, gazed outside and saw to my horror that we had stopped outside the house of the V**. Surely – surely – I thought, Em does not live here. Next moment, Mistress had opened my private car door and was encouraging me to jump out. I dug my feet in and refused to oblige. I have never yet entered the V**'s house without having to suffer and I didn't see why I should go in now. But Mistress, as you know, has an Iron Will. She grabbed my collar, pulled it hard and said, "Stop being so silly, Hamish." So, of course, I had to go in.

A beautiful spring day had turned from joy to pain.

The V**'s house had its usual scent of anxious dogs and miserable cats. I was made to stand on a table. Master, to his credit, stroked my head, while I looked reproachfully at him. The V** prodded and poked in his heartless way. He stuck a needle in my neck, felt my ribs, then took a narrow tube and ... no, I refuse to remember what he did with that tube. Finally, he said, "Hmm, Hamish is a bit overweight but he has passed his Em o' Tee."

Now, finally, I understood: "Em o' Tee" wasn't a person after all, but a process – a rather nasty kind of dog examination, at the end of which I had been declared "a bit overweight". I glared hard at the V**. I foresaw – correctly – a bleak future, where I was deprived of all bones and biscuits until I regained my proper, slim whippet profile.

So, yes, today is a beautiful spring day. I am older now, and wiser. There is joy, joy, joy in the heart of a silver brindle whippet with a white stripe down his nose. The grass is a juicy green. There is a whiff of daffodils and young rabbit in the air, et cetera, et cetera, et cetera.

But the wiser, older Hamish now says to himself: if spring has come, can Em o' Tee be far behind?

11

Release

In the western world, we are rich beyond measure in material terms – even the poorest citizen has a material quality of life that the poor of the developing world can only dream of. For 55 years I had enjoyed good health and access to health care on the few occasions I required it. Even working amongst the direst poverty as a volunteer teacher in Africa, I had usually had the basics of food, water and reasonable security. In the UK, I always had enough income to live well, where "well" equals having a secure roof over one's head, friends, family, interesting job, stimulating social life and enough to eat and drink. This post-stroke world was teaching me to savour each of these things more fully and carefully.

And now I was about to re-enter fully into that world.

The first snow of the winter had fallen during the night. There was a damp, cold feel to the day as I hobbled stiffly with Jo through and out of the automatic doors from the Woodend stroke unit. It was Friday 19 November 2004, almost exactly four months since I'd been wheeled into Akershus Hospital in Oslo. I had progressed to the extent that I could limp heavily about, a splint strapped to my left leg and my left arm held tightly across the front of my body. I eased myself slowly into the passenger seat of our car, carefully following a procedure I'd been instructed in by the occupational therapists.

A few days earlier Botox injections had been administered in the underside of my forearm, and the growing tension in the fingers of my left hand was already beginning to ease. Botox – botulinum toxin – treatment can be used on patients to reduce excessively high tone in stroke-affected muscles. I had laughingly suggested that it could also be used to improve my beauty, but I didn't laugh for long, because the procedure had not been quite as painless as promised. The consultant had used the opportunity to demonstrate this relatively new procedure to nursing and other medical colleagues. I lay tensely on my back on a plinth surrounded by them. An electric current was passed through each muscle which was to be injected, causing the relevant finger to flex and bend and my lower arm to feel as if it was on fire. I'd glanced briefly at the needle and thereafter kept my eyes focussed slightly to the right so that I could not actually see him manoeuvring it into the correct position. Four injections and a series of electric currents later I was ready to deliver a severe verbal beating to the nurse who'd told me that this was a simple, painless procedure. I knew she would respond by calling me a wimp.

As I sat in the car waiting for Jo to return from the ward with one or two items, I could feel that my wrist and fingers were not pressing so firmly against my stomach. I felt ill and tired and my face felt tight in the cold air, but at least I was leaving behind the deadly routine of hospital life and entering the comparative freedom of home.

I had fantasised about home for weeks. I had visualised going from room to room, simply enjoying the comfort of the familiar furniture, the photos and pictures on the walls. Above all, I'd fantasised about silence when I wanted it, with company and noise when I chose to have it, and the absence of loud, trashy television.

The reality, of course, was different.

A few weeks before discharge from Woodend, I was released to spend weekends at home. At this time, I was still confined to a wheelchair, and so we'd prepared for the two major obstacles this seemed to present: the two shallow steps at our front door and the main staircase to our bedrooms. The first was to be overcome by two parallel ramps up which the wheelchair could be pushed. The second would be overcome by restricting me to the ground floor. This would be fine as we had a toilet and wash hand basin downstairs. What I'd forgotten was the sheer quantity of furniture that had to be negotiated as I "furniture walked" around using my good arm for support. When you are able bodied, you think nothing of deftly bypassing a low table to get to a chair. When your leg feels like a dead weight, there's a constant ache in your buttock, every step is an effort, you are horribly nauseous and perpetually threatening to overbalance, that low table becomes an immense threat and challenge. The sheer effort of moving about exhausts and dispirits.

The physiotherapists had warned me against attempting to walk because it immediately raised the tone in my arm, causing it to flex and press against my stomach. Nevertheless, I was determined at least to negotiate my way to the toilet on my own. Each time I felt the slightest twinge in my bladder, I would wind myself up in preparation for the journey from my seat in our sitting room to the toilet located below the staircase in the hallway. Thoughtful occupational therapists had already provided a raised toilet seat and raised feet had been inserted under one of our armchairs. The house was beginning to acquire the accoutrements of an old folks' home. I determined that, as soon as possible, these physical signs of bodily weakness and decline would be returned to sender, that the house would resume the appearance of a normal home.

Over the first few days of my permanent return home Jo and I settled into a routine. I was still confined to the downstairs rooms. Having gone to bed, exhausted, by about 7 p.m., we'd waken early. Jo would shower and take Hamish for a walk. If she wakened earlier than me, which she often did, she would slip into the kitchen for a quiet cup of tea with yesterday's newspapers or the current book. To begin with, there were weekly visits from the physiotherapist and occupational therapist. For much of the day I sat motionless, exhausted and nauseous, or listened to books on CD.

After a couple of weeks we had an additional handrail installed on the staircase and I was finally able to crawl stiffly upstairs and sleep in my own bed. This also had the huge advantage that I could have a proper bath – downstairs, I had been restricted to a bowl of soapy water.

In the mornings, Jo would connect the bath chair controls, leave a towel for me and encourage me to get up. I would always lie in bed for a few minutes, testing my left side for signs of improvement. I would postpone the actual moment of standing up for as long as decently possible. When I lay in bed, on my back, it was possible to believe for a few glorious minutes that I was whole again. I felt normal. If I shut my eyes, I could imagine walking in the nearby countryside with Hamish trotting along close by. Once I stood up, my left side immediately became tense and painful. My left buttock would ache and my foot press hard into the carpet. I'd spend the rest of the day following exercise routines suggested by the physiotherapists, reading, sleeping and delighting in only watching such television as I chose. Walking outside was confined to brief forays into the garden close to the house.

I discovered when I returned home that friends had helped Jo to keep on top of house and garden while she expended all her energy on travelling to Woodend and visiting me. I wept with gratitude on learning this. Emotionally I was still a hopeless mess – I would scream in frustration, yell and cry with self-pity. Jo stood serenely by but I suspect she was anything but serene in reality.

Eventually, after some weeks, physiotherapy and occupational therapy ceased. I was told by medical staff that long-term physiotherapy for stroke patients "could not be afforded." If I wanted more physiotherapy to aid further recovery, I would have to pay for it myself. Jo and I were on our own to face the rest of this together.

12

The Constancy of Dog

There are some days when I wonder if life is worth-while.

I had this feeling a few weeks ago when I awoke one morning to discover that the very soul had been ripped from my life. My jaw dropped as I stared from my kitchen-bed across the room to the space where the heart of my life, the centre and meaning of my existence, the epicentre of all my fantasies had previously lain, reliably and constantly for as long as I can remember. I am referring, of course, to the small circular bowl which houses my food, and the little tin dish which holds my water. The bowl and dish had vanished! Gone. Vamoosed.

We whippets, like most dogs, appreciate certainty, and that bowl and that dish had been securely housed in the same spot for years – a cosy, sheltered niche close to the tempting cooking smells of the kitchen, but nicely private and sheltered from the comings and goings of Master and Mistress. But now, some human – no dog would have done this – had removed them and replaced them with a large sterile white box which hummed quietly. Of bowl and dish there was not a trace to be seen.

Even as I began to digest this appalling information, Mistress swept into the kitchen and began banging plates on a table. As is my custom in the early morning, I leapt out of bed, padded across the room and rubbed my head up and down against her leg. I find that this helps to remind her of my existence and my undying affection. It also helps to let her know that it is time I was given some food and drink – oh, and love, too, of course. Who can resist an early morning rub from a rather handsome silver-brindle whippet, with a manly white chest, velvety ears and a white stripe down his nose? Well, actually, Mistress can. Her loving response to my morning rub was "Yes, yes, Hamish. I know you're there." And she carried on banging plates on the table.

This left unanswered the question of what had happened to my food bowl and water dish. Was I to be left to starve? I went over to the humming white box, saw that a metal tray had been placed next to it, and began to rattle this as hard as I could. I hoped this would alert Mistress to the fact that my universe was changed, changed utterly.

Mistress' reaction was decisive.

Her hand was instantly round my collar, dragging me in the direction of the back door and there ... there ... in the draughtiest spot in the whole of our home ... there, just beside the door, were the bowl and dish, awaiting my attention. As usual, the bowl contained a bare sufficiency of dry food, and the dish a skim of water. So, the message was clear – from now on, Hamish, faithful loving family dog, was to take his modest meals next to the chill draught of an outside door, displaced from the old comfortable eating niche by a mysterious white, humming box.

But worse was to come.

As she walked away from me, Mistress opened the front of the white box. A great cloud of freezing air blew out from it. She stretched her hand inside, withdrew a little frozen box, then closed the door again. I was puzzled. Why would Master and Mistress move my bowl and dish to the most inconvenient spot in the house and replace it with a useless white box, which, as far as I could see, contained lots of frozen air and a couple of chilly little packages?

I did not have to wait long for an answer.

Master breezed in, put his arm around Mistress and said, "Oh, yes. This is going to be far more convenient than fetching frozen food from the garage." Then he stood back, looked admiringly at the white box, glanced at me and added: "Don't you think so, Hamish?"

I gave Master a bleak look of disapproval – the truth had dawned on me at last. My food and dish had been displaced to make life more convenient for Master and Mistress. In order that they didn't have to walk the very short distance from house to garage for their sumptuous scoff, I was to take my meagre meal exposed to the gusts of cold air round the back door.

As I say, sometimes I wonder if it is all worthwhile – but I know I won't complain. I'll just get on with it and soon that chilly spot at the back door will be the centre of all my future food-related fantasies.

But, then, that's the infinite adaptability and constancy of dog.

13

Bogarn

Bogarn, our home in Glen Dye was surrounded by beautiful, forested countryside, but it was out of reach for now – the rough tracks were beyond my weak faltering body.

By late March 2005, and several sessions of private physiotherapy at a Sports Centre in Aberdeen, I was beginning to feel greater normality in my left leg. I still bobbed to the left, walked stiffly with a stick and I still felt as though the leg could collapse beneath me, but the constant ache in my buttock and knee was beginning to diminish. There was a regular meeting in the sports centre for stroke survivors of all ages and conditions which was run by the charity Different Strokes. This is a charity that exists to provide support for younger stroke survivors and contact with them opened my eyes to how relatively fortunate I had been in terms of physical damage following the stroke.

However, again I found myself asking the question – Is this the best we can do as a wealthy, civilised country to provide long-term health care for stroke survivors? At the time of writing we have a Scottish government in place with a forward-looking policy on acute in-patient stroke care, but little to say about the long-term health care entitlements of stroke patients when they leave hospital. We also have a Scottish government whose policy – I quote the words of the then Minister for Public Health – is to "drive private providers to the margins of the NHS". Yet, it is currently these same maligned "private providers" who offer the only hope of long-term treatment for stroke survivors. It was a superb private physiotherapist who finally got me more fully mobile – what is to happen to those who cannot afford this treatment? Time, I think, for a more grown-up debate between politicians and the public about the relationship between independent health providers and the NHS. A frank admission by politicians that a publicly funded health service cannot hope to provide every aspect of health care that our society requires would be a start.

I had my final appointment with the consultant at the end of March 2005. I had been trying to manage without the splint attached to my leg, but he strongly advised wearing it once again. He urged me not to think of this as taking a step back but as a way of ensuring that the leg and foot remained correctly aligned. Head could see the sense of this but heart felt as it had back in September when the idea of wearing a splint was first broached. I resumed using it and immediately heart felt vindicated as my toes began curling tightly whenever I tried to walk. Each day I would walk stiffly one hundred metres or so down our driveway to the road and back again. My toes would curl tightly and painfully against the gentle downward slope of the road. Some time later I would walk back up again, my knee snapping backwards each time I straightened my left leg.

I had a twice daily routine of stepping up and stepping down on to a small plinth left by the physiotherapist and by the second half of April I was able to do three sets of ten of each steps without feeling utter exhaustion and dizziness.

Gradually, gradually over months and years, milestones were noted and passed. I was allowed to drive again. I resumed work, in a small way at first then more fully and more confidently. I was able to travel independently away from home. And every day, I walked.

Each day I would hobble up a track through the woods. For months, my left leg felt stiff, leaden and useless. My left arm, tight and painful, was fixed rigidly at a right angle in front of me. I clasped a walking-pole in my right hand. The clumsy plastic splint, strapped to my left leg, lurked uncomfortably beneath loose trousers. Each day I would push myself a little further. I would note the tree – pine or birch or fir – to which I had managed to struggle, panting and exhausted, before returning home.

On each trip, I would scream to the sky.

At night I'd lie awake in bed thinking of those trees – silent, impassive sentinels of my progress, imagining their softly rustling shadows under a starry northern sky, waiting for my return next day.

Those trees were a small pleasure and a subtle, healing balm.

14

Anniversary

Anniversaries are the memory hooks where, for good or ill, we hang the treasures of our lives – births, love affairs, marriages. Deaths. Strokes.

Each day is an anniversary for David. We remember him quietly in our hearts. His life flows through us. He is never far away. We mention his name as often as possible. Each birthday – 2 July – we place flowers on his grave. Each 28 September we remember his death in life. Each Christmas, we raise a glass to him. Each New Year we enter another year without him, another year in which his potential will never be fulfilled.

But today it is not New Year; today is not a day of special birth or death; it is not a day for riotous celebration; but it is an anniversary of a kind, the fourth anniversary of a life saved to fight another day.

It is a warm but breezy mid-July. The full-leaved trees blow and rustle in hot woodland waves. The man parks his aging Volvo estate at the top of the track which leads in a gentle slope to the river. With an effort, grasping the side of the vehicle, he climbs out. He walks to the rear, raises the tailgate and a silver-brindle whippet leaps delicately out.

The man picks up a walking pole, looks for a moment at it, then replaces it in the rear of the car. The whippet trots along the track, occasionally glancing back at the man. The dog's face has a white stripe and a mournful expression. The man locks the car, and slowly follows the dog along the track. The man's gait is slow, hesitant and slightly unsteady, but together they keep going for a quarter mile or so until they reach the river. The dog sniffs around for a bit, occasionally holding his head up into the breeze.

Together they spend long, long minutes gazing at the dark river where it flows rapidly past a small shingle beach.

Acknowledgments

I am grateful to all the medical professionals who treated me in Norway and the UK, to John Forster for his invaluable help in commenting on the text of this book and to Jo, with whom everything is possible.

Some of Hamish's musings first appeared as a series of articles in *The Deeside Tattler*, a magazine edited by Aboyne-based musician and composer, Sheila Maxwell, on behalf of the Scottish Episcopal churches of upper Deeside.

Several stroke charities in the UK undertake tireless work to raise awareness of stroke, to support stroke survivors and to fund research into stroke. They include:

The Stroke Association
www.stroke.org.uk

Chest, Heart and Stroke Scotland
www.chss.org.uk

Different Strokes
www.differentstrokes.co.uk

Lightning Source UK Ltd.
Milton Keynes UK
UKOW05f0619190617
303652UK00001B/7/P